Table o

ENERGY SMOOTHIES
Energizer Smoothies
Supreme Smoothie
Mango and Peach Smoothie
Cocoa and Peanut Butter Smoothie
Coffee Smoothie

SUPER FOOD SMOOTHIE
Berry Smoothie
Beetroot Smoothie
Orange and Flax Seed Smoothie
Banana Nuts and Cocoa Smoothie
Avocado and Coconut Smoothie

MEMORY BOOSTER SMOOTHIES
Berry Medley
Dates and Walnuts Smoothie
Cantaloupe and Raw Egg Smoothie

CLEANSE SMOOTHIES
Go Green Smoothie
Green Smoothie
Best Cleanse Smoothie
Kale Smoothie
Detoxifying Smoothie

LOW SUGAR/DIABETIC SMOOTHIES
Diabetic Smoothie
Low Carb Green Smoothie
Diabetic Oatmeal Smoothie
Pineapple and Spinach Smoothie
Peach Smoothie for Dietetics

DESSERT SMOOTHIES

Apple Dessert Smoothie
Caramel Smoothie
Key Lime Yoplait Smoothie Recipe
Peanut Butter Smoothie
Oreo Smoothie

DAIRY FREE SMOOTHIES

Sunshine Smoothie
Granny Smith Apples Smoothie
Banana and Nuts Smoothie
Pineapple and Avocado Smoothie
Soymilk Smoothie
Cocoa and Macadamia Smoothie

KETOGENIC SMOOTHIES

Peanut Butter Caramel Milkshake
Blueberry Smoothie
Blackberry Chocolate Smoothie
Cherry Vanilla Smoothie
Keto Strawberry Milkshake

HIGH PROTEIN SMOOTHIE

Pomegranate and Beetroot Smoothie
Raspberry Almond Chia Smoothie
Peanut Butter and Jelly Smoothie
Green Banana Smoothie
Very Berry Smoothie

SMOOTHIES FOR GOUT & ARTHRITIS

Smoothie to Help with Gout
Kiwi and Kale Smoothie
Melon-Mango Smoothie
Strawberry-Orange Smoothie
Grapefruit Smoothie

BEST SMOOTHIES BY BLOOD TYPE

Smoothie for Type A Blood Type
Smoothie for Type B Blood Type
Smoothie for Type AB Blood Type
Smoothie for Type O Blood Type

Energy Smoothies

Energizer Smoothies

Prep Time: 4 Minutes
Servings: 6

Ingredients

- 2 gala apples, skin and seeds removed
- 2 cups almond milk
- 2 tablespoons of crushed almonds
- ½ teaspoon of cinnamon powder
- 2 teaspoons of crushed walnuts
- 1 teaspoon of almond butter
  Ice cubes, for chilling

Directions

1. Blend all the ingredients in a high-speed blender for 40 seconds.
2. Serve in smoothie glasses.
3. Enjoy chilled.

Supreme Smoothie

Prep Time: 5 Minutes
Servings: 6

Ingredients

- 2 mangoes, peeled and pits removed
- 4 ripped bananas, peeled
- 2 cups milk
- 2 green apples, seedless and cubed
- Ice cubes, for chilling
- 1/3 cup mint leaves, for garnishing

Directions

1. First wash all the fruits thoroughly.
2. Then peel the bananas and place it in a blender.
3. Next, peel and remove the pit of mangoes and dump the pulp into the blender.
4. Then add in the seedless apple chunks and mint leaves.
5. Pour in the milk.
6. Pulse until combined.
7. Pour into serving glasses.
8. Enjoy chilled.

Mango and Peach Smoothie

Prep Time: 5 Minutes
Servings: 6

Ingredients

- 2 mangos, peeled and diced
- 2 peaches, fresh and cubed
- 1/3 cup pumpkin seeds
- ½ cup almonds
- 2 cups of almond milk
- 1 cup ice cubes, for chilling

Directions

1. Combine all the listed ingredients in a blender and pulse until smooth.
2. Serve into glasses and enjoy.
3. Enjoy chilled.

Cocoa and Peanut Butter Smoothie

Prep Time: 6 Minutes
Servings: 7

Ingredients

- 2 cups almond milk, unsweetened
- 2 tablespoons of peanut butter, natural and organic
- 1 tablespoon of almonds, unsweetened
- 4 tablespoons of cocoa powder, unsweetened
- 3 tablespoons of honey
- 2 cups of ice cubes

Directions

1. Pour all the listed ingredients into a high-speed blender.
2. Blend for 30 seconds.
3. Once smooth, pour into serving glasses and enjoy.

Coffee Smoothie

Prep Time: 5 Minutes
Servings: 2

Ingredients

- 2 tablespoons of organic coffee beans
- 1 cup plain milk
- 2 tablespoons of flaxseed meal
- Ice cubes, for chilling
- 1 cup cold water, for brewing the coffee
- 2 tablespoons of brown sugar

Directions

1. Grind the coffee beans and brew the coffee in the brewer.
2. Next, pour the brewed coffee into the high-speed blender and add milk, flax meal, ice cubes, and sugar.
3. Blend for 30 seconds.
4. Pour it into the tall glasses.
5. Serve and enjoy immediately.

Super Food Smoothie

Berry Smoothie

Prep Time: 5 Minutes
Servings: 4

Ingredients

- 1 cup cranberry juice
- 4 strawberries, fresh
- 1 cup blueberries
- 1 cup Greek yogurt
- 4 tablespoons honey
- 1 cup crushed ice

Directions

1. Blend all the listed ingredients in the high-speed blender.
2. Once the smooth consistency is obtained, pour into glasses and enjoy.

Beetroot Smoothie

Prep Time: 5 Minutes
Servings: 2

Ingredients

- 2 cups fresh pineapple, chunks
- 2 cups Beetroot, washed
- 1 cup kale
- ½ teaspoon of lemon juice
- 4 tablespoons of honey
- 2 cups of ice cubes

Directions

1. Combine all the listed ingredients in the high-speed blender.
2. Pulse it for one minute.
3. Once the desired consistency obtained, pour into tall serving glasses.
4. Serve and enjoy.

Orange and Flax Seed Smoothie

Prep Time: 5 Minutes
Servings: 4

Ingredients

- 2 cups peaches, sliced
- 2 carrots, juice only
- 2 cups orange juice
- 2 tablespoons ground flax seeds
- 1-inch fresh ginger, chopped
- 2 gala apples, seedless and skinless
- 1 cup ice cubes for chilling

Directions

1. Combine all the listed ingredients in the blender.
2. Pulse it for 40 seconds.
3. Once the smooth consistency is obtained serve in tall glasses and enjoy.

Banana Nuts and Cocoa Smoothie

Prep Time: 5 Minutes
Servings: 4

Ingredients

- 2 cups of almond milk
- 4 bananas, ripped and peeled
- 1/3 cup of walnuts
- 1/3 almonds, chopped
- 2 tablespoons of honey
- ½ cup dates pits removed
- 2 teaspoons cocoa powder
- 1 cup ice cubes, for chilling

Directions

1. Peel the bananas and remove the pits from the dates.
2. Take a blender and combine all listed ingredients in it.
3. Blend for one minute at high speed.
4. Once the smooth consistency is obtained, serve into tall serving glasses and enjoy.

Avocado and Coconut Smoothie

Prep Time: 5 Minutes
Servings: 6

Ingredients

- 3 avocados, fresh and pitted
- 1 tablespoon of coconut oil
- 3 cups coconut milk
- 2 tablespoons of coconut flakes
- 1 teaspoon of sugar
- Ice cubes, for chilling

Directions

1. Pulse all the listed ingredients in a high-speed blender for one minute, until a smooth consistency is obtained.
2. Pour into serving glasses.
3. Enjoy.

Memory Booster Smoothies

Berry Medley

Prep Time: 5 Minutes
Servings: 4

Ingredients

- ½ cup strawberries
- 1 cup blueberries
- 1 cup raspberries
- 2 cups coconut milk
- 1 cup crushed ice cubes
- 1 tablespoon flax seeds

Directions

1. Combine strawberries, blueberries, raspberries, flax seeds and coconut milk in a blender.
2. Pulse it for 50 seconds at high speed.
3. Now add ice cubes to serving glasses and pour the smoothie into it.
4. Serve chilled and enjoy.

Dates and Walnuts Smoothie

Prep Time: 5 Minutes
Servings: 2

Ingredients

- 1 ripe banana, peeled
- 4 dates, pitted
- 1 tablespoon raw almond butter
- 1 tablespoon raw cacao powder
- ½ cup walnuts, grounded
- Ice cubes, for chilling

Directions

1. Blend all the listed ingredients in the high-speed blender.
2. Pour into tall smoothie glasses and enjoy.

Cantaloupe and Raw Egg Smoothie

Prep Time: 5 Minutes
Servings: 4

Ingredients

- 1 organic large egg, beaten lightly
- 1 cup Cantaloupe, fresh
- 2 teaspoons of sesame oil
- 2 cups milk
- 2 tablespoons of honey
- 1 teaspoon of flax seed
- Ice cubes, for chilling

Directions

1. First, blend egg in a blender until foamy.
2. Then add cantaloupe melon and oil.
3. Pulse it for a few seconds.
4. Next add milk, flax seeds, honey and ice cubes.
5. Blend it until smooth in consistency.
6. Next, pour it into serving glasses.
7. Enjoy.

Cleanse Smoothies

Go Green Smoothie

Prep Time: 4 Minutes
Servings: 3

Ingredients

- 2 carrots, peeled
- 4 cucumbers, peeled
- 1 cup parsley
- ½ cup of baby spinach
- 1 cup kale
- 1 lime, squeezed
- 1 cup water, filtered
- Pinch of salt

Directions

1. Wash all the vegetables before start making the smoothie.
2. Cut all the vegetables into small chunks.
3. Place all the vegetables with remaining listed ingredients into the high-speed blender.
4. Pulse it for 30 seconds.
5. Pour into serving glasses.
6. Serve and enjoy chilled by adding ice cubes.

Green Smoothie

Prep Time: 5 Minutes
Servings: 4

Ingredients

- 2 cups coconut water, cold
- 1 cup greens, roughly chopped
- A handful of parsley
- A handful of cilantro
- 1 cucumber, diced
- 6 green apples, cored and diced
- 1 cup diced peaches
- Ice cubes, for chilling

Directions

1. Add all the listed ingredients into the high-speed blender.
2. Pulse it until smooth.
3. Pour into the serving glasses.
4. Enjoy.

Best Cleanse Smoothie

Prep Time: 5 Minutes
Servings: 5

Ingredients

- 1 stalks kale, stem removed
- 1 cup baby spinach
- 1 lemon, seeds removed and peeled
- 1-inch ginger, peeled
- 1 cucumber, peeled and diced
- A Handful of fresh parsley
- 6 pears, chopped
- 2 green apples, seeds removed
- 2 cups water
- Ice cubes, for chilling

Directions

1. Add all the listed ingredients into the high-speed blender.
2. Pulse it until smooth.
3. Pour into the serving glasses.
4. Enjoy.

Kale Smoothie

Prep Time: 5 Minutes
Servings: 6

Ingredients

- 1 cup cherries
- 2 cups of kale, stem removed
- 2 cups water
- 4 teaspoons of hemp seeds
- 1 cup ice cubes
- 1/3 cup blueberries

Directions

1. Add all the listed ingredients into the high-speed blender.
2. Pulse it until smooth.
3. Pour into the serving glasses.
4. Enjoy.

Detoxifying Smoothie

Prep Time: 5 Minutes
Servings: 4

Preparation Time: 5 Minutes
Yield: 5 Servings

Ingredients

- 1 apple, peeled, de-seeded and cubed
- 2 cups grapes
- 4 sticks of celery
- 2 cups kale
- Ice cubes, for chilling
- 1 cup water

Directions

1. Add all the listed ingredients into the high-speed blender.
2. Pulse until the desired consistency is obtained.
3. Pour into tall serving glasses.
4. Enjoy chilled.

Low Sugar/Diabetic Smoothies

Diabetic Smoothie

Prep Time: 5 Minutes
Servings: 4

Ingredients

- 1 cup strawberries, chopped
- 1 cup unsweetened almond milk
- 1 cup Greek-style yogurt, low fat
- 1 cup ice cubes, for chilling

Directions

1. Place all ingredients in a blender.
2. Pulse until the desired consistency is obtained.
3. Pour into tall serving glasses.
4. Enjoy chilled.

Low Carb Green Smoothie

Prep Time: 5 Minutes
Servings: 4

Ingredients

- 1 cup water
- 1 gala apple, cut into cubes and seeds discarded
- 1 green pear, cut into chunks
- 2 cups spinach
- 20 Moscato grapes
- 2 tablespoons agave nectar, or to taste
- Ice cubes, for chilling

Directions

1. Place all ingredients in a blender.
2. Pulse until the desired consistency is obtained.
3. Pour into tall serving glasses.
4. Enjoy chilled.

Diabetic Oatmeal Smoothie

Prep Time: 5 Minutes
Servings: 5

Ingredients

- 1 cup uncooked oats, grounded
- ½ ripe banana, peeled
- 3 cups almond milk, unsweetened
- 2 tablespoons of ground flax-seed
- 4 teaspoons of stevia
- 2 teaspoons of coffee extract

Directions

1. Combine all ingredients in a high-speed blender and pulse for 30 seconds
2. Pour into tall serving glasses and enjoy.

Pineapple and Spinach Smoothie

Prep Time: 5 Minutes
Servings: 4

Ingredients

- 1 cup water
- 1 cup pineapple, chunks
- 2 cups baby spinach
- ½ cup celery sticks
- 1 green apple, chopped and seeds removed
- 1 tablespoon of stevia, to taste
- Ice cubes for chilling

Directions

1. Add all the listed ingredients into the blender.
2. Pulse until a smooth consistency is obtained.
3. Pour into the ice-filled serving glasses.
4. Enjoy.

Peach Smoothie for Dietetics

Prep Time: 5 Minutes
Servings: 4

Ingredients

- 1 peach, peeled, pitted, and chopped
- 1 cup plain milk
- 1 cup Greek yogurt
- 1 cup ice cubes
- ½ teaspoon of ground cinnamon, or to taste
- 2 scoops of stevia, or to taste

Directions

1. Place milk, peach Greek yogurt, ice cube, stevia and cinnamon in the blender.
2. Pulse it until smooth.
3. Pour into serving glasses and enjoy.

Dessert Smoothies

Apple Dessert Smoothie

Prep Time: 5 Minutes
Servings: 2

Ingredients

- 1 cup of apples, stewed
- 1/3 teaspoon of cinnamon powder, or to taste
- ½ cup of vanilla ice cream
- 2 oatmeal cookies, crumbled
- 1 cup milk

Directions

1. Place all ingredients into your blender.
2. Blend for a few seconds until all ingredients combined into a smooth consistency
3. Pour into ice-filled serving glasses and enjoy.

Caramel Smoothie

Prep Time: 5 Minutes
Servings: 4

Ingredients

- 1 cup whole milk
- 1 scoop of chocolate ice cream
- 1 scoop of vanilla ice cream
- 2 tablespoons of dark chocolate chips, unsweetened
- 1 tablespoon of butterscotch sauce
- Handful of peanuts

Directions

1. Place milk, chocolate ice-cream, vanilla ice-cream, chocolate chips, butterscotch sauce and peanuts into your blender.
2. Blend for a few seconds until all ingredients combined into a smooth consistency.
3. Pour into ice-filled serving glasses and enjoy.

Key Lime Yoplait Smoothie Recipe

Prep Time: 5 Minutes
Servings: 2

Ingredients

- 1 cup fat-free Key lime pie yogurt
- 1 ripe banana, sliced
- ½ cup organic milk
- 1 tablespoon lime juice
- 1/4 teaspoon of dry lemon lime-flavored soft drink powder
- 1 cup vanilla frozen yogurt

Directions

1. Pulse all ingredients except frozen yogurt into your high-speed blender.
2. Pour into tall ice-filled servings glasses.
3. Serve with a dollop of frozen yogurt on top.

Peanut Butter Smoothie

Prep Time: 5 Minutes
Servings: 4

Ingredients

- 3 frozen bananas
- 1 tablespoon cocoa powder
- 1 tablespoons peanut butter
- 1 cup almond milk
- 1/3 teaspoon vanilla extract

Directions

1. Add all the listed ingredients into the blender.
2. Pulse it until smooth.
3. Serve into glasses and enjoy.

Oreo Smoothie

Prep Time: 5 Minutes
Servings: 1

Ingredients

- 1 cup Vanilla ice cream
- ½ Cup Milk, low fat
- 7 Oreo cookies, crushed

Directions

1. Add all the listed ingredients into the blender.
2. Pulse it until smooth.
3. Serve into glasses and enjoy.

Dairy Free Smoothies

Sunshine Smoothie

Prep Time: 5 Minutes
Servings: 4

Ingredients

- 2 cups coconut milk
- 4 bananas, peeled, sliced
- 1 cup of mango, flesh
- 1 cup strawberries
- Ice cubes for chilling

Directions

1. Combine all the listed ingredients in a high-speed blender.
2. Blend until smooth.
3. Serve and enjoy.

Granny Smith Apples Smoothie

Prep Time: 5 Minutes
Servings: 4

Ingredients

- 1 cup spinach, washed
- 1 cup kale
- 4 granny smith apples, peeled and cored
- 1 cup purified water

Directions

1. Place all the listed ingredients in a blender.
2. Blend until smooth.
3. Serve into glasses and enjoy.

Banana and Nuts Smoothie

Prep Time: 5 Minutes
Servings: 4

Ingredients

- 1/3 cup of walnuts, crushed
- ½ cup almonds, crushed
- 1 cup oats, soaked overnight
- 1 cup of almond milk
- 2 bananas
- 4 dates, pitted
- Ice cubes, for chilling

Directions

1. Combine all the listed ingredients in your blender.
2. Pulse it until smooth.
3. Serve into glasses and enjoy.

Pineapple and Avocado Smoothie

Prep Time: 5 Minutes
Servings: 4

Ingredients

- 1 cup pineapple
- 2 avocados, cored and peeled
- 2 cups coconut milk
- Ice cubes, for chilling

Directions

1. Combine all the listed ingredients in a high-speed blender.
2. Blend until smooth consistency.
3. Serve into glasses.
4. Enjoy.

Soymilk Smoothie

Prep Time: 5 Minutes
Servings: 4

Ingredients

- ½ cup almond butter
- 1 cup strawberries
- 1 cup soy milk, unsweetened
- 1 cup ice cubes

Directions

1. Combine all the listed ingredients in a blender.
2. Blend until smooth consistency is obtained.
3. Serve into tall glasses and enjoy chilled.

Cocoa and Macadamia Smoothie

Prep Time: 5 Minutes
Servings: 4

Ingredients

- 2 tablespoons of honey, or to taste
- 4 tablespoons macadamia nuts, crushed
- 1 tablespoon of cocoa powder
- 2 cups coconut milk
- 1 cup ice cubes

Directions

1. Add all the listed ingredients in a blender.
2. Pulse it until smooth.
3. Serve in smoothie glasses and enjoy.

Ketogenic Smoothies

Peanut Butter Caramel Milkshake

Prep Time: 5 Minutes
Servings: 3

Ingredients

- 1 cup ice cubes
- 2 cups coconut milk, unsweetened
- 4 tablespoons peanut butter
- 4 tablespoons Salted Caramel
- 1 teaspoon **xanthan gum**
- 2 tablespoons **MCT oil**

Directions

1. Add all the listed ingredients in a blender.
2. Pulse it until smooth.
3. Serve in smoothie glasses and enjoy.

Blueberry Smoothie

Prep Time: 5 Minutes
Servings: 4

Ingredients

- 2 tablespoons **flaxseed meal**
- 2 tablespoons **Chia seeds**
- 2 cups unsweetened coconut milk
- Few drops of stevia
- ½ cup blueberries
- 2 tablespoons **MCT oil**
- ¼ teaspoon **xanthan gum**

Directions

1. Add all the listed ingredients in a blender.
2. Pulse it until smooth.
3. Serve into ice-filled smoothie glasses and enjoy.

Blackberry Chocolate Smoothie

Prep Time: 5 Minutes
Servings: 2

Ingredients

- 1 cup coconut milk
- ½ cup blackberries
- 1 tablespoon of cocoa powder
- Few drops of stevia
- 1 teaspoon of xanthan gum
- 1 cup ice cubes

Directions

1. Add all the listed ingredients in a blender.
2. Pulse it until smooth.
3. Serve in smoothie glasses and enjoy.

Cherry Vanilla Smoothie

Prep Time: 5 Minutes
Servings: 4

Ingredients

- ½ cup full-fat canned coconut milk
- ½ cup water, filtered
- 1/6 teaspoon pure vanilla powder
- Sea salt, pinch
- 1 cup organic sweet cherries
- 1 cup ice cubes

Directions

1. Add all the listed ingredients in a blender.
2. Pulse it until smooth.
3. Serve in smoothie glasses and enjoy.

Keto Strawberry Milkshake

Prep Time: 4 Minutes
Servings: 4

Ingredients

- ½ cup coconut milk
- ½ cup heavy whipping cream
- Ice cubes, for chilling
- 2 tablespoons Strawberries
- 2 tablespoons MCT oil
- 1/3 teaspoon xanthan gum

Directions

1. Add all the listed ingredients in a blender.
2. Pulse it until smooth.
3. Serve in smoothie glasses and enjoy.

High Protein Smoothie

Pomegranate and Beetroot Smoothie

Prep Time: 5 Minutes
Servings: 4

Ingredients

- 1 cup beet-root, peeled
- 1 cup Greek yogurt
- 1 cup pomegranate juice
- 2 teaspoons honey
- Ice cubes, for chilling

Directions

1. Add all the listed ingredients into the blender
2. Blend for 30 seconds.
3. Once the desired consistency obtained, pour into tall glasses and enjoy.
4. Serve and enjoy.

Raspberry Almond Chia Smoothie

Prep Time: 5 Minutes
Servings: 4

Ingredients

- 1 cup plain Greek yogurt
- 2/3 cup almond milk
- ½ cup raspberries, frozen
- 1/4 cup almonds, divided
- 2 tablespoons honey
- 1 tablespoon of Chia seeds

Directions

1. Add all the listed ingredients in a blender.
2. Pulse it until smooth.
3. Serve in smoothie glasses and enjoy.

Peanut Butter and Jelly Smoothie

Prep Time: 5 Minutes
Servings: 4

Ingredients

- 1 cup of non-fat Greek yogurt
- ½ cup almond milk, unsweetened
- 2 scoops stevia
- 25 green grapes
- ½ cup peanut flour
- Ice cubes, for chilling
- 1 tablespoon of protein powder

Directions

1. First, add Greek yogurt, almond milk, stevia, and grapes in a blender.
2. Pulse it for a few seconds.
3. Then add peanut flour, protein powder, and ice cubes.
4. Pulse until a smooth consistency is obtained.
5. Enjoy.

Green Banana Smoothie

Prep Time: 5 Minutes
Servings: 4

Ingredients

- 1 large banana, peeled, frozen
- 1 cup Greek yogurt
- 1 cup almond milk, unsweetened
- 2 cups baby spinach
- 1/3 teaspoon vanilla extract
- 2tablespoons almond butter
- 1 teaspoon of protein powder

Directions

1. Add all the listed ingredients in a blender.
2. Pulse it until smooth.
3. Serve in smoothie glasses and enjoy.

Very Berry Smoothie

Prep Time: 5 Minutes
Servings: 4

Ingredients

- 2 cups water
- 2 cups spinach
- 2 cups mixed berries, frozen
- ½ cup yogurt
- 2 scoops vanilla protein powder
- 1 tablespoon of walnuts, grounded
- 1 teaspoon of flaxseed, grounded

Directions

1. Add all the listed ingredients in a blender.
2. Pulse it until smooth.
3. Serve in smoothie glasses and enjoy.

Smoothies for Gout & Arthritis

Smoothie to Help with Gout

Prep Time: 5 Minutes
Servings: 4

Ingredients

- 1-1/2 cup of water
- 1 cup pineapple, cubed
- 1 orange, peeled and deseeded
- 1 carrot, chopped
- 1 tablespoon Chia seeds
- 1-inch fresh ginger
- Handfuls of baby spinach

Directions

1. Add all the listed ingredients into the blender.
2. Pulse it until smooth.
3. Serve into glasses and enjoy

Kiwi and Kale Smoothie

Prep Time: 5 Minutes
Servings: 4

Ingredients

- 1 cup of water, filtered
- 2 mangoes, peeled and pitted
- 2 kiwi fruits, peeled
- 1 cup kale, torn into pieces

Directions

1. Pulse all the ingredients in a blender until smooth.
2. Serve into ice-filled glasses and enjoy.

Melon-Mango Smoothie

Prep Time: 5 Minutes
Servings: 4

Ingredients

- 1 cup of filtered water
- 1 cup cantaloupe, cubed
- 2 mangos, peeled and pitted
- 4 large strawberries
- 2 cups baby spinach, washed

Directions

1. Pulse all the ingredients in blender until smooth
2. Serve into ice-filled glasses and enjoy.

Strawberry-Orange Smoothie

Prep Time: 5 Minutes
Servings: 4

Ingredients

- 1 cup of filtered water
- 2 bananas, peeled and sliced
- 6 strawberries
- 2 oranges, de-seeded
- Ice cubes, for chilling

Directions

1. Pulse all the ingredients in a blender until smooth.
2. Serve into ice-filled glasses and enjoy.

Grapefruit Smoothie

Prep Time: 3 Minutes
Servings:4

Ingredients

- 1 cup filtered water
- 1 fresh banana, peeled and sliced
- 1 red grapefruit, peeled and seedless
- 1 cup pineapple, cubed
- ½ cup fresh parsley

Directions

1. Pulse all the listed ingredients in a high-speed blender for one minute.
2. Pour into ice-filled serving glasses.
3. Serve and enjoy.

Best Smoothies by Blood Type

Smoothie for Type A Blood Type

Prep Time: Minutes
Servings: 4

Ingredients

- 2 scoops Protein Blend Powder A
- 1 cup water
- ½ cup soy milk
- 1 cup of blackberries

Directions

1. Pulse all the listed ingredients in a high-speed blender for one minute.
2. Pulse until a smooth consistency is obtained.
3. Pour into ice-filled serving glasses.
4. Serve and enjoy.

Smoothie for Type B Blood Type

Prep Time: 5 Minutes
Servings: 4

Ingredients

- 1 cup strawberries
- 1 banana
- ½ cup low-fat yogurt
- 1 cup milk
- 1 cup grape juice
- 3 teaspoons honey

Directions

1. Pulse all the listed ingredients in a high-speed blender for one minute.
2. Pulse until a smooth consistency is obtained.
3. Pour into ice-filled serving glasses.
4. Serve and enjoy.

Smoothie for Type AB Blood Type

Prep Time: 5 Minutes
Servings: 2

Ingredients

- 4 carrots, peeled
- 1 cup grapes
- 1 cup rice milk
- 4 tablespoons of Agave syrup, or to taste
- 1 cup ice cubes, for chilling

Directions

1. Place all ingredients in a blender.
2. Pulse until the desired consistency is obtained.
3. Pour into tall serving glasses.
4. Enjoy chilled.

Smoothie for Type O Blood Type

Prep Time: 5 Minutes
Servings: 4

Ingredients

- 2 scoops Protein powder
- 1 cup water
- 1 cup almond milk
- 1 ripe banana, peeled
- 1 cup of blueberries
- 1 cup cherries
- ½ cup pineapple, cut into small chunks

Directions

1. Combine all the listed ingredients in a blender.
2. Pulse it until smooth.
3. Serve into ice-filled glasses and enjoy.
4. Enjoy chilled.

Made in the USA
Las Vegas, NV
27 June 2025

24157729R00042